My Baby Lives

A True Story
By
Erika Lopez

My Baby Lives

I dedicate this book to my Lord and Savior Jesus Christ, my amazing husband, my best friend Rafael Lopez, and my sister, Vivian Gonzalez, who was always by my side, and always told me I can do all things, and of course, Santiago Beato—the baby that lived, and the reason behind this book.

My life is a product of so many God has sent along the way as angels to get me through.

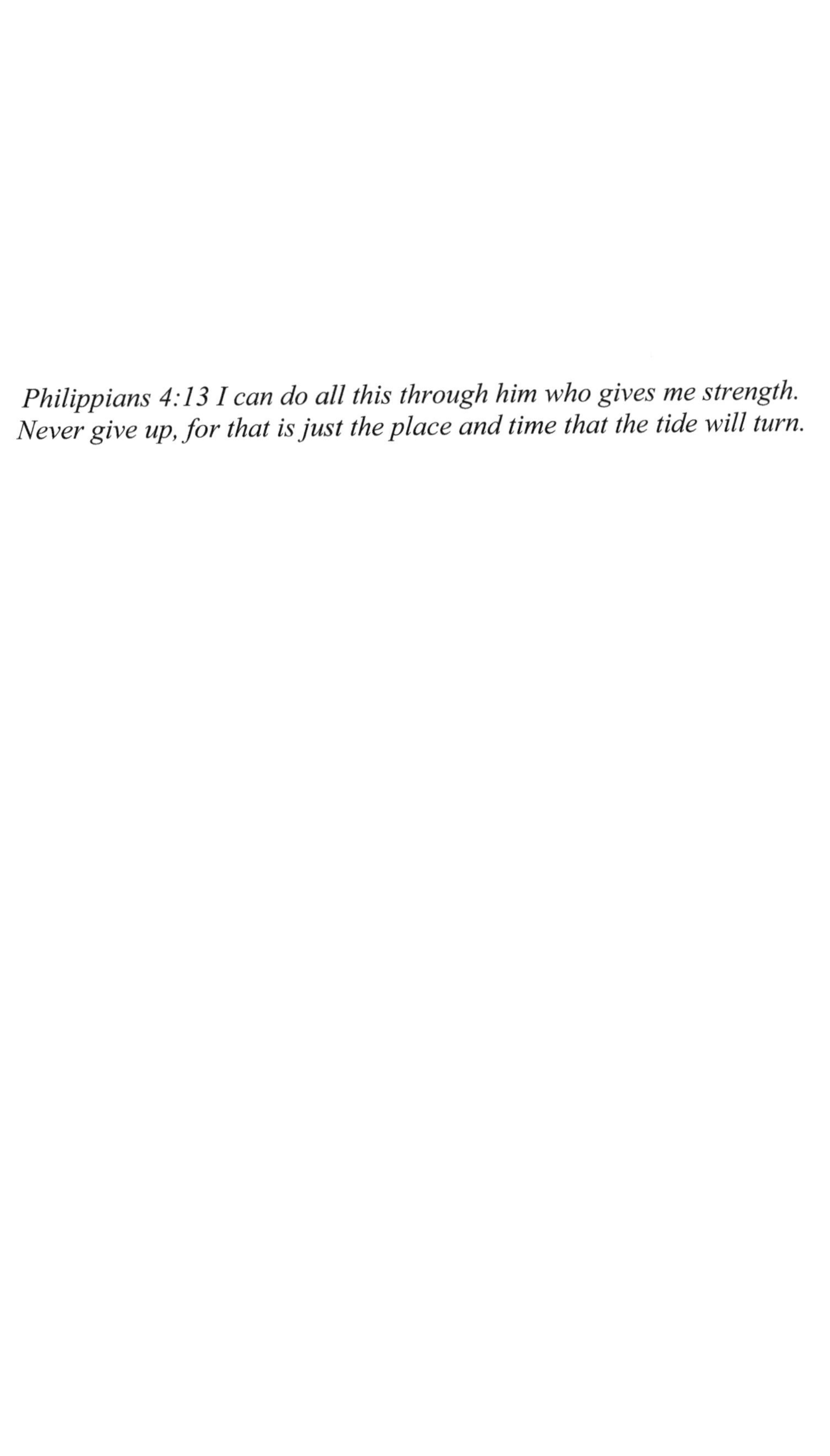

Philippians 4:13 I can do all this through him who gives me strength.
Never give up, for that is just the place and time that the tide will turn.

May we always support life not only the life in the womb, but let's support the lives of moms and dads. Family has always been a God plan. Choose life today!

"Now listen! Today I am giving you a choice between life and death, between prosperity and disaster. 1 For I command you this day to love the Lord your God and to keep his commands, decrees, and regulations by walking in his ways. If you do this, you will live and multiply, and the Lord your God will bless you and the land you are about to enter and occupy

Deuteronomy 30:15-16

Today, by the grace of God, I have decided to embark on a journey to tell my story. The story I hope will inspire other girls, and also to share the trials that I know many others face each day.

My faith has led me to heal, and also to rejoice even in my sufferings because they have built endurance and perseverance in my life. I've learned to trust and to be patient, and I know love conquers all. I choose today not to give up on life, but a hope for a greater future by knowing that you can achieve all things if you set your mind to it. I've learned not to live life in fear, but to live a life filled with faith, and this faith has given me hope for the future.

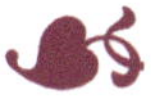

Life is a journey clothed with many different experiences, and many we can't explain. But each piece of clothing sets small parts of our life. I like to see it as clothing because it's something you can change. The great mistake we sometimes make is that we keep wearing the same clothing into the other seasons of our life, causing us to not be able to change.

This is a story of a young girl filled with fears and emotions that were unexplainable.

You ever feel a certain way, but don't know why? It all began when she was so young girl. So afraid but not knowing what fear even was.

She held her breath at night when she heard sounds, but did these sounds even exist? The very thought of getting up at night to use the restroom caused panic and anxiety. She bit her nails till they bled. The thought of another day and having to be in a school or surrounded by people felt too scary to imagine. Her dad would hold her hand outside the restroom door. This was the only way she would go. Mom would stand outside the little glass at school so she could make it through the day. The moment the face disappeared pure panic arose. Lunch breaks at school were the worst when hundreds of others roamed the hallways. What if they came near and what if they wanted to speak to her?

Fear is an unexplainable feeling—whether you're afraid of heights or animals. Fear causes major limitations and keeps us from who and what we should be.

Maybe these fears began in a family that practiced witchcraft or maybe the nightmares caused the fears to increase throughout the day. There is no way to know, but this little girl was a very frightened one.

As time passed, having one friend was enough to help calm the fear of being at school—to know someone else was there brought great comfort. When the seasons changed and life began to progress, friends came in and out of her life. They didn't realize how much more they were needed. Whatever she needed to do to be wanted and accepted was a possibility. After being sheltered in private school and not being able to leave her mom's side, something huge happened. Dad decided to move to start a new job in a faraway place—at least, that's what it seemed like.

She had finally grown up a bit and became comfortable with the daily routines of school and dance life. Who would want to start over? She was only nine years old and felt like life was a horror movie. What else could go wrong? Oh, I know let's put her in a public school—the place we spoke of that people got beat up at and bad people went to, at least, that's all she knew. Fear creeped in greater than before. She worked hard at being sick every morning. This sickness was far from fake—it was a sickness that progressed and got worse as the months went by.

Thankfully, after a couple of months, she made a friend that wasn't exactly the best role model, but it helped shape her fears and teach her how to get by in this new season and begin a new journey.

The Journey of Acceptance Began

MY BABY LIVES

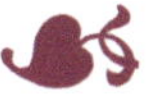

Who would have known she would have met the man of her dreams at thirteen. Most of her dreams were nightmares, but this fictional story of acceptance seemed wonderful. There was a boy that needed her and told her how pretty she was. He was a bad boy that was always in trouble. Trouble sounded fun at that point. She was just a good girl looking to be loved and protected. Her friend taught her how to dress and how to act so that she could be accepted and never left alone. Why would a bad boy want a good girl? "Just pretend to be someone you're not," her friend told her.

That's when the great pretending began. Sometimes we don't realize we begin to clothe ourselves with things we should not wear. Fear and being a pretender was not who she was meant to be, but who was she? I don't think she had any idea. She was just a sheltered little girl filled with fear and now pretending to be a girl she knew nothing about. "Make sure you tell this boy you are not a virgin. Boys don't want a good girl virgin because they don't want to get stuck with them."

After months of pursuing this journey, cutting school and hanging out in parks and visiting empty homes, this life seemed like the best life ever. It felt like freedom! Soon, the great moment arrived. She was invited to his home. What a cool place! Everyone was there and everything seemed so fun. He had his own room with a big lock on the door. When that door locked, the fear kicked in, but this life was way better than what she felt before.

The magic question arose, "Are you a virgin?"

"Of course not," she replied, "I've been with lots of people."

I don't think he quite believed her. He told her, "I don't want to be with you if you're a virgin." I think he noticed she was pretending to be someone she was not. But she insisted she was not a virgin, and it was ok.

That day she entered a new world—a world she had no idea about. She never learned the story of the birds and the bees—maybe just the story of purity. She wanted to be loved and protected. This seemed like the answer for sure now. He gazed at her face after lying with her, and said, "You were a virgin. I'm sorry what have I done." But I think he felt something he had longed for as well—someone who thought you were the best person ever had to be a major gift. She was only fourteen, and he was barely sixteen. Both were not very experienced with life, and both had no role models who could show them the way. Well, the ones they had they wouldn't want to share these mistakes with. But life felt good, and waking up to the very thought of being together was the best feeling ever.

Shortly after our events and many visits together, it turned out she wasn't the only girl experiencing these feelings. Girls he said he had nothing to do with chased and threatened to hurt her. He expressed how he wanted her and only her because she was his good girl. Wow, her friend was right. Guys get stuck with good girls, but how would he know how to treat her?

She shortly learned that this life was more fearful than the one she had before. What if she lost him? What if one day he didn't want her or what if he chose someone else instead of her? All those terrible thoughts crossed her mind, and fear crippled her to love him more than anything. No matter what he did or said it was okay.

She knew he loved her. He promised he would be with her no matter what. He would tell her she was the "pearl in the oyster."

The Great Unexpected

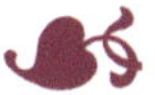

The great unexpected happened. She found out she was pregnant. How would this work out? How would she tell her parents? All these questions filled her mind. Here was a little girl trying to make decisions based on no knowledge of what to do. Her parents didn't even know she was in a relationship. She absolutely lied about everything, and this boy never existed in their minds. Of course, her friend had the answer, "Don't tell no one, not even him and I will take you to Planned Parenthood in the morning." Just get rid of the baby and pretend this never happened."

What? I hadn't heard of this place, or how it even worked. Her mind was lost for thoughts of aborting a baby and even more lost to think that she couldn't share this with the person she felt that she loved more than anything in the world, but fear of the unknown crippled her. What would her mom say and what would he say? Would he even want a baby or maybe he would just leave her. She thought she had become nothing but a problem.

It was early in the morning when she skipped school and went to the clinic with her friend. They tested her again and then placed her in a room to meet with a counselor. As she waited in the room for someone to come in, the minutes felt like hours. Soon as sweet woman walked into the room and I began to cry. She began to explain to me the options and explained that I was safe and didn't have to tell my parents about the visit.

Option one was that I could have an abortion. I'd always heard of them. I went to catholic school all my life, and I knew couldn't do that. But, at this moment, it sounded like the easier choice. She began to explain how easy and simple it would be. All I needed to do was make another appointment and come in. They would give me a pill, and shortly after, it would all be over. All I remembered was crying. I don't know what the other option was—they never shared it—but I did know I didn't want to face my mom. I was so afraid.

I went ahead and scheduled my next appointment. My friend was waiting for me outside in the lobby. We walked out of that place, and she encouraged me that I had made the right decision. The next week was my appointment, but the night before something inside of my heart and inside of my belly told me not to do this, but I didn't know what else I *could* do. There I was at the appointment. I filled out some paperwork and was taken into a room. I was told to change into a gown and sit on a table in the room. I was so afraid and crippled by the thoughts of what would happen next. They took a sonogram but didn't let me see it and explained the next steps. Then they left the room and informed me that the nurse would be in shortly. I quickly got off the table and put my clothes back on and told them I wanted to leave. They wanted me to meet with the counselor first. Once again, I still had not taken this pill. They told me I had to take it, and at this point I didn't want to. I was afraid, but more than anything, I knew I had just seen a baby inside of me. I was already sixteen weeks pregnant.

I called my boyfriend in complete desperation. I told him I had to meet him right away, and that I had something to share with him. We would always sit outside in front of his building. When I told him I was pregnant, he asked me by who. I began to cry, thinking he didn't believe me. Then he looked at me with a scared look on his face. We were two scared people trying to figure it out. We sat outside and held each other. I cried and he told me everything was going to be ok. I knew he felt bad for me. I told him I went to have an abortion, but I couldn't do it. He promised not to leave me and that he would do whatever he could to help me.

Early the next morning, I had to tell my mom. This was getting more real by the minute. I wasn't brave enough to tell her face to face, so I wrote a letter. My mom would wake up early every day and would shower and lay her clothes out on the bed. It seemed like a great idea to just put the letter under her clothes and leave for school. When she went inside the bathroom, I snuck in her room and put the letter under her clothes. Then I tiptoed out and went to school.

My dad would drive me to school and back. Silence was the best word to describe that morning drive. Every minute in school felt like an hour as I waited for my mom to arrive. I pictured she would show up and pull me by my hair out of the classroom or come get me and take me back to that clinic. The time had come. The intercom went off calling my name to the office and when I arrived, my father was there to pick me up. He told me my mom didn't go to work and that she needed to speak to me. He seemed confused and didn't know why. I didn't know what would happen next. It was a long silent ride home. Maybe my mom would throw me out or maybe she would make me have that abortion or maybe she would just beat me till I miscarried. These where all the thoughts that went through my mind on the way home.

As I arrived home, my mom asked my dad to leave and told me to sit down. The first question that came out of her mouth was, "What are your plans?" As the letter stated, she already knew I went for an abortion and couldn't follow through with it. I said I didn't know what to do. She said it seemed like I'd already made a choice to be an adult. She asked me what I was going to do. I told her I wanted to have my baby. She asked me about the boy and how old he was. The disappointment in my mother's eyes made me feel even worse, but now we had to tell dad. I loved my dad so much. I couldn't imagine disappointing him. What would he think of his little girl?

Life went on. Dad didn't speak much to me through the pregnancy, actually he hardly spoke to me at all, but it was clear what an embarrassment I was to the family. Babies having babies was the famous quote from everyone. I began to prepare. I had a crib in my room, and all kinds of things that my mom bought for my new baby. The time had come, and my mom and boyfriend were at the hospital with me after fourteen hours of excruciating pain. They decided to give me medication to induce labor. My boyfriend couldn't even be in the room, and all he kept saying was I'm so sorry I did this to you. He couldn't face all the pain I was going through.

I gave birth to a beautiful baby boy. He was the light of my life. 6 lbs. 9 oz. I held him as if it were the most precious thing in the world, well, he was to me, and still is. The thought of sleeping without him in my arms was impossible, but the next day he had a high fever, and they didn't understand what was going on. After bloodwork, they realized I had an infection in my body. They took the baby from me and told me I wouldn't be able to touch him until they could figure out what was wrong and put me on antibiotics. For the first time, my dad had come to the hospital. I think he thought I would die. He told me he loved me, and that everything was going to be okay. Wow. That was amazing! I hadn't heard my dad's voice in seven months!

I got better. They discharged me and I went home with my beautiful baby boy. I took pictures every moment of the day. For the first time ever, I felt like I had a purpose. That purpose was to raise a child—meaning making sure he always had everything he wanted or needed. He also needed love and protection. As I looked in his eyes, I realized he wasn't afraid like I was. He felt safe in my arms.

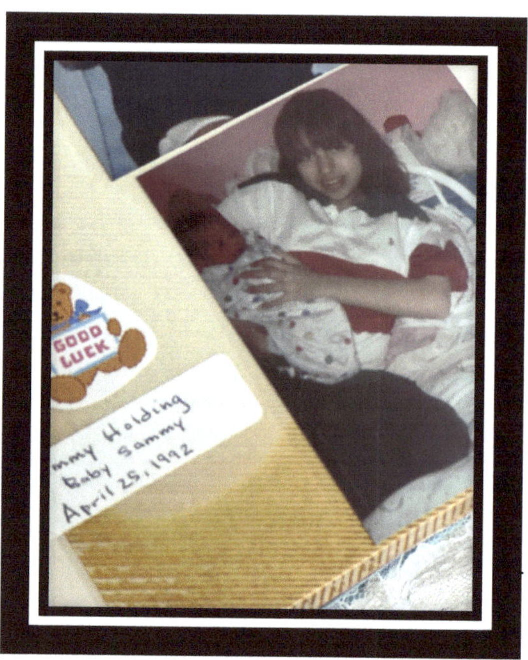

Season Changed Quick and Women-hood Began

A journey as a mom.

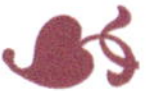

I wasn't sure what Mom meant, but I knew it was the best feeling I had ever felt. This little boy that looked at me depended on me. His life was in my hands. No matter my age, it was time to grow up. How could I hold the life of a person that I loved with a love I had never felt before? The world taught me that parents take care of their children. But where would I begin? I was only fifteen years old. I couldn't even take care of myself. I couldn't get a job either. Problems at home got worse and my mom and dad were always fighting. My dad would throw me out of the

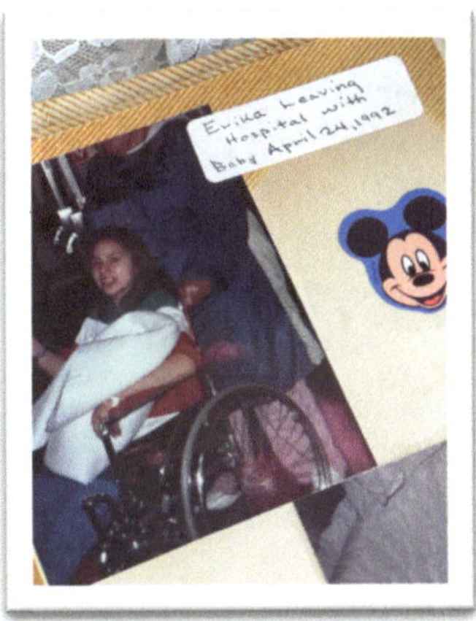

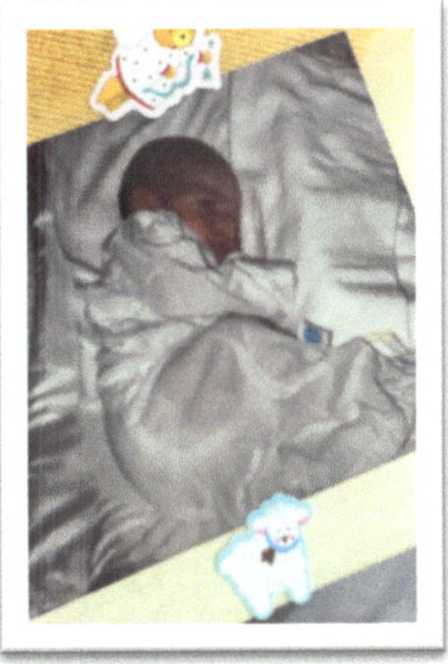

house every day. I don't know if he meant it or not, but I knew that I hated the feeling of not having security.

My boyfriend decided that he would talk to his mom about me moving in over there with the baby. She agreed, and life changed drastically. I started a new life that I never knew. They were very poor.

I didn't know what it was to live without an air conditioner at the window. The first time I told him I was really hot, he went and got a bucket of water with a towel and put it on my chest. We had a small room in his mom's apartment and there we slept with an antenna on the TV and rags on ourselves to stay cool. It definitely was not the life I knew.

Well, there began my journey into the system that could help me. I didn't know much about welfare and never visited one of their offices. My father always took care of me. Both my parents worked all my life. I found myself standing in a long line and waiting a long time at social services only to be told after waiting eight hours that I had to go to another office. This place was scary. I was afraid, had no money, and was hungry. I remember wishing I could buy a hotdog at the hotdog stand outside the office and maybe even a drink, but I didn't have money for that. I was desperate to figure out how my world was going to work out. The people that were in my life knew how to work the system very well, so they began to teach me what I needed to say and how I needed to say it so that I could get the support I needed.

Crazy how desperate people live. When I look back now, with tears falling on the page of this paper as I write, I realize how we can live our life in survival mode only to live each day to survive.

After all the hard work, I finally got some answers. I was given insurance so that I could go to the doctor and paperwork that I had applied for services so that I could now begin to look for an apartment, but nobody told me that they only give you enough for housing that nobody wants—housing a spoiled little girl like me never knew even knew existed, but I finally found a place. My friend's mom had introduced me to a landlord that owned lots of buildings. I went to visit this alleyway apartment. It wasn't the nicest place, but it was only five hundred a month. I thought how I could make it my own, and little by little make it nicer and nicer. But the exciting thing was that I could move in with my boyfriend and my baby.

I received the apartment and did exactly what I had planned. I began to clean it. My friends gave me things and helped me make it nice. That place was scary. My dad lived on the other side of town, but he had walkie-talkies that he used, and he said that I could get a signal and stay connected with him. I slept with a walkie-talkie underneath my pillow. Now that I think about it, it wouldn't make sense if someone had broken in because it would have taken him so long to get to me, but it still made me feel safe knowing I could contact him.

Having a young boyfriend that always wanted to hang out in the streets, I was always alone. I never knew where he was. Some days he never came home. Life wasn't what I expected it would be, but it was *my* life.

The apartment was roach-infested and filled with mice, but all I cared about was having a place where I could take care of my baby. I had a family that lived next door to me—a woman who lived with her boyfriend and had five kids in a small little apartment like mine, but this lady became my savior. She was like a mother to me and grandma to my baby. She would help me with everything. She taught me how to cook and would check up on me often. She would even buy me groceries with the little bit she had and took me to stores with her. I will never forget her. Her name was Rosa.

Rosa taught me how to catch the mice. She would put strings across my sink at night and fill the sink with water and Clorox. Crazy to even think about it now. I never imagined something like that existed. Everything was a learning experience, but the crazy thing is I actually really loved my life. Rosa taught me how to take care of plants I still have till this day. She was in an abusive relationship and sometimes I would hear her scream. I knew I couldn't help her, but I was afraid for her.

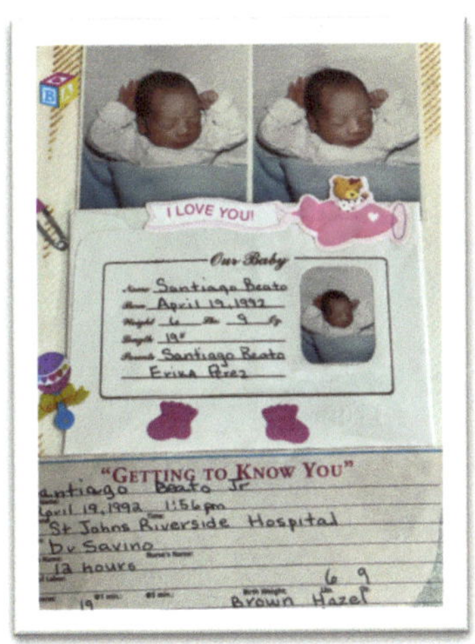

I found myself not having enough to pay the bills. What would I do? How could I get money for clothing and things we needed to survive. I decided to begin to look for a job and lying was the only way to make this happen, so I created a fake birth certificate so I could work. I worked hard only to find out that I no longer would be given the money for my rent from welfare because I had a job. How would I survive off my work pay and pay rent? I was slowly losing everything.

Soon, I had to start over. I landed a job at Payless Shoe Store, and I worked really hard there. My mom agreed to watch the baby. At just fifteen years old, I worked forty hours a week to make enough money to pay all my bills. My hard work led to me getting a great position as an assistant store manager. Who would've thought a 15-year-old girl could do such a thing? I was determined to take care of my baby, but never really got to see him at this point, but I was proud—proud when I came home, proud to carry him, proud to buy him stuff. I slept holding him really tight. Fear was all I knew—fear of someone or something hurting us.

MY BABY LIVES

Years began to go by and jobs kept coming. I changed jobs and changed homes a lot, but things kept getting better. I kept working—I kept fighting doing what I knew was best. My son never lacked anything. I even got married. We went to city hall and my dad and boyfriend's mom signed since we were too young.

Time and years went by with so many losses and disappointments. I began to get weary and tired but never told anyone. I even thought of not wanting to live, but who would take care of my baby if I didn't? So, I kept on getting up and pushing through.

In 2009, for the first time I turned to something that I was told would help me stay awake and help me work harder. I thought no person could hold you back if you could provide for all your needs. That wasn't true. I found myself trying drugs for the first time and once again I started to lose everything. How many times do you fight? How many times do you restart? No one tells you this.

I remember when everyone told me to be pro-life and to never get an abortion because God will punish you. There were so many reasons why I kept my baby, but once he was born, help was hard to come by. I found myself realizing that God had brought me through time and time again And I began to look to him—not to help me, but for him to take my life.

I tried to take my life. It was one pill that led to more pills. These pills almost ruined my life in one year. I knew I was about to lose everything I worked so hard for. My house was in foreclosure, and my car was about to get repossessed. But all I could think about was a pill and how I could get another one. I was filled with shame and anger towards myself, and that's when I decided to do it.

How did I get to this place? And what do I do now? I took not one but an entire bottle of Vicodin and a bottle of Ambien. I was hoping to lose this battle. That I would never wake up again as I fell asleep. I didn't stay there. I woke up in the arms of my boyfriend. My boyfriend who never prayed but found a way to pray to God that I wouldn't die. He prayed that if God saved me, we would find a way to live for him.

I woke up. God finally answered a prayer. This prayer changed my life forever. I got saved. The road of life didn't get easier, but it did have a purpose. Now that I'd found Jesus, I found a friend I was always looking for. I found a helper—someone who could help me when I didn't know what to do. It was what I had always dreamed of. Why hadn't anyone told me how good this life could be if I had just known Jesus? Why didn't someone help me besides just telling me that he existed? Why didn't someone help me know him better?

He began putting people in my life fifteen years ago, and now God has been the author of my story. Now I realize he was with me every step of the way. He was the one that always made a way for me even when I didn't know him. He was always there. He was the one who protected me in that dark alleyway apartment. He was the one that kept me alive.

I'm so happy I lived to tell the story of my life for me and my child. This child was never a mistake. He was the *purpose* why God gave me life. God showed me true love through him. He showed me how to fight and not give up. And when I couldn't fight no more, he stepped in and became Lord of my life and fought the battle for me. Salvation came when I learned how much he loved me. God showed me character and challenged me on the trials and tribulations.

Healing was slow, but God began from the inside of me. Troubles never ended, trials only got bigger, but shame never popped in my mind again I knew that God had changed my life and made me the mom I am today. He had a plan even with all the shame and hurt.

MY BABY LIVES

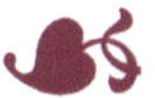

I watched my son making the same mistakes as I was building my dream life with God. My son began to do the very things that hurt my life. He began to drink and use drugs. I began to fight this battle on my knees praying for my son by loving him and making sure that I told him every day about how special he was.

Somehow, I was able to pretend this wasn't reality. I just saw him as the perfect child of God that I loved. I prayed, I cried, I hoped, and God heard my prayers. God writes our story, no matter what mistakes we make. God can make a way where there is no way.

Me and my family live our life with our hope in the Lord. We've learned to trust him during very trying times. We've learned to stand together, support each other, help each other, and keep our hope in the Lord—the one who is in control of all things.

My son is thirty-years old today, and currently a youth pastor. He loves his family and his children. I have two grandchildren that he's given me; my baby Bethel (five), and Judah (two). I also had three other children; a beautiful daughter named Seleste, who is now twenty-six years old and serves the Lord, and she's married to her amazing husband. She has three beautiful children; Winter (five), Summer (three), and our newest edition, baby boy Zion who is three-weeks old today.

In 2020 after fostering for three years, we adopted Apollo Paul. He has blessed our life and taught us unconditional love in a whole new way.

My wonderful husband, Rafael Lopez, has lived through my healing journey and stood by me every step of the way. We are now married and have been for twelve years now. He has become an amazing father to all my children, even the two that he stepped in to take care of. I love him and I can say I'm living the dream now. We both serve the Lord. We have many dreams that we still have not lived out here on earth, but one we live for the most is to help other people. We love to find those that are lost –those that are hurting, because I know if we could help someone and make their life a better place on earth, we can show them who Jesus is through our character.

I don't want to just tell women not to have an abortion, I want to tell them like I told Apollo's mom. If you have him and can't take care of him, I will help you. It wasn't the easiest decision, but we ended up staying by our word. Everyone who says they are pro-life should be willing to lay down their own life for the sake of another child or offer help to the mother who wants to raise her child on her own.

You can change the world. God has given us the ability to love each other. Love comes from God. It's an action that must live through our lives and everything we do. Love isn't just a word—it's a commitment to be there for each other. Let's build families, not only with those related to us, but with those who God puts in our life that we could inspire.

I am also the mother of a special needs child who is now twenty-years old. God has given me the grace to love him and raise him to know Jesus. The battle of having a special needs child is not easy, and I am still looking for the solutions on how to build a network where Moms can get the help they need.

When I think of all the needs in our world for children, I wish I could make them all come true—from an orphanage that will love children—to churches and networks around the world who will make a place for moms to be able to bring their children with special needs and behavioral issues.

All the time I find moms who struggle to find a proper setting for their children. Pro-life is bigger than just telling people they should not kill their babies, pro-life is about a baby and a mother. It is also building families that will come alongside mothers. Especially when we tell them they should have their special needs child and that having an abortion is murder. Who will rise up and buy diapers and help with housing and childcare? Who will rise up to watch your child when mom just needs a break?

I will. I decided to write this story as a mother who still asks these questions every day, but has not given up the fight, and now I know that the Lord is the one who gives me strength. I want to live to encourage others through the body of Christ to help and equip each other to be the people God says we could be.

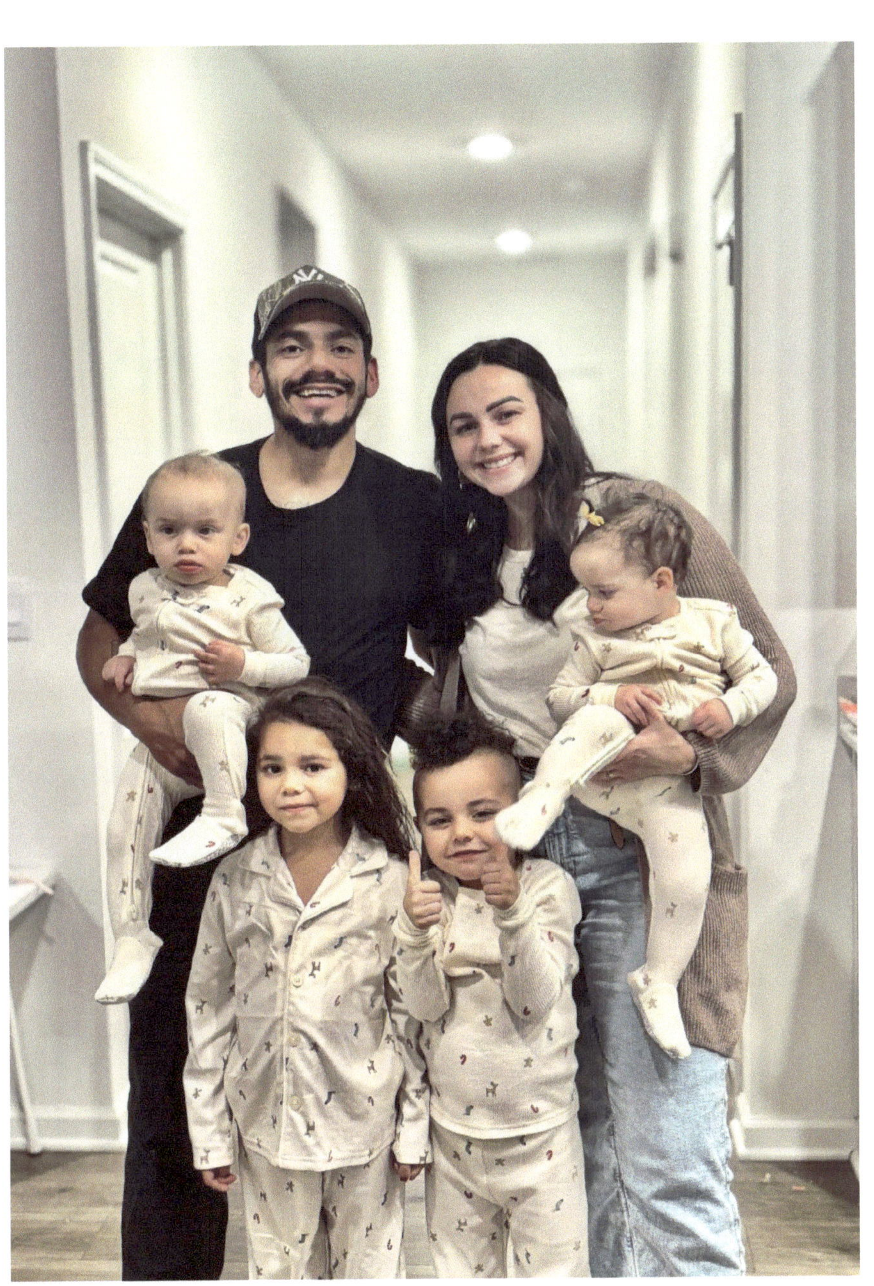

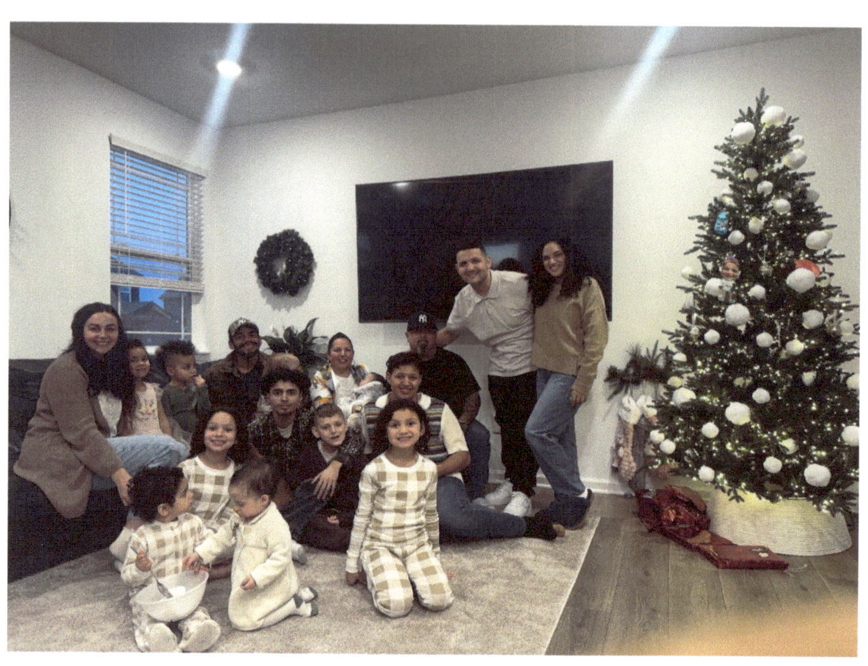

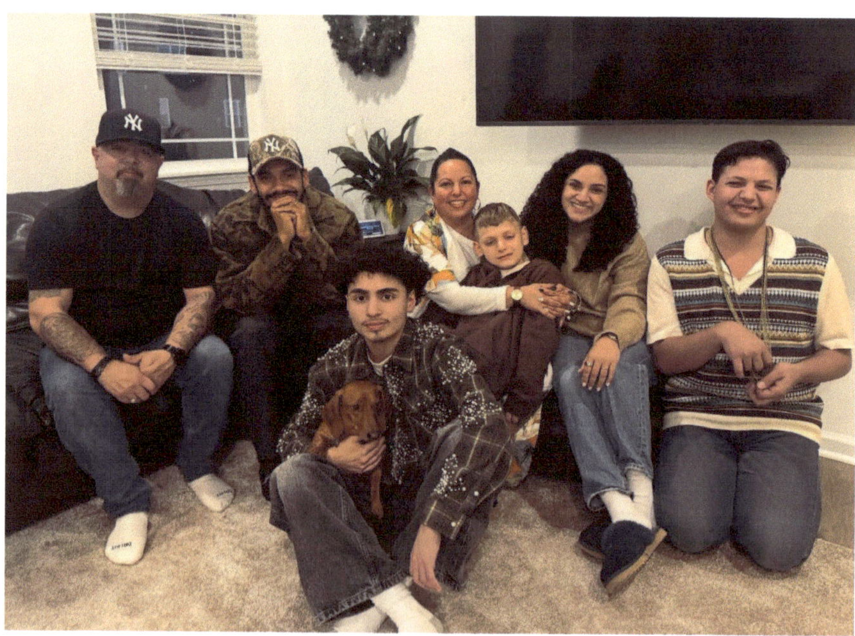

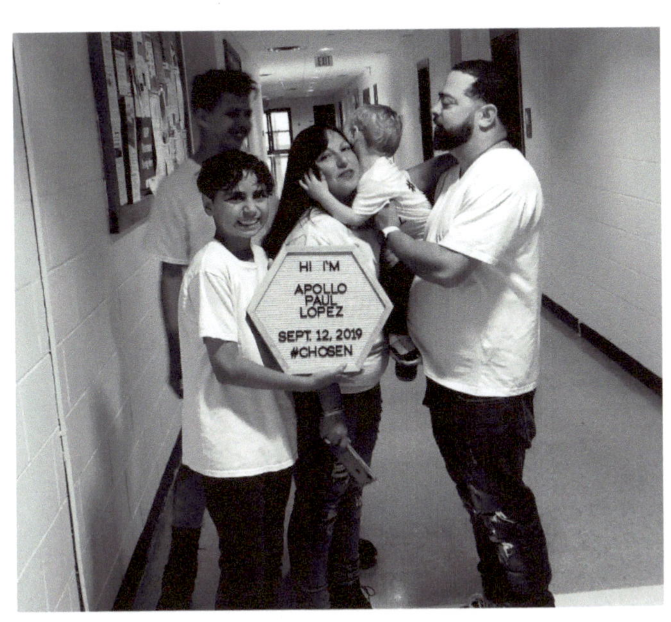

HI I'M
APOLLO
PAUL
LOPEZ
SEPT. 12, 2019
#CHOSEN

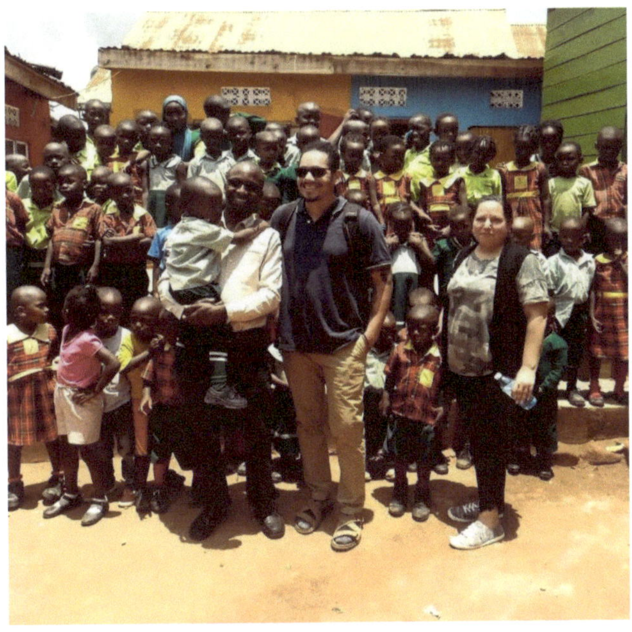

Erika Lopez a wife of her, Amazing Husband , Rafael Lopez, and mother of five children, grandmother of five grand-babies, Pastor and most of all a messenger as service, Jesus Christ. She loves to love people and share the love of Christ.

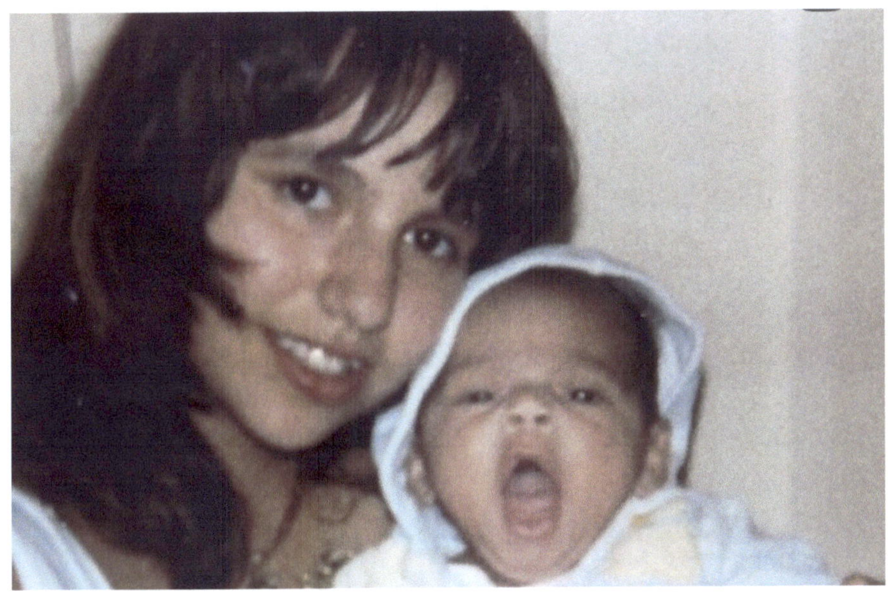